LIVING 120 YEARS
THE SECRETS TO EXTENDED LONGEVITY

www.chobanu.com

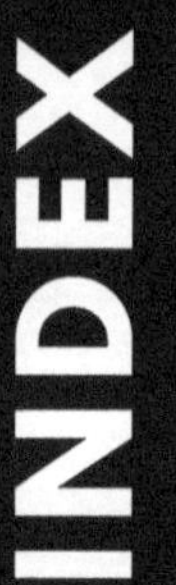

INDEX

Is it possible to live for more than 120 years?

According to the Guinness World Records, Jiroemon Kimura from Japan was the oldest man ever. He lived for 116 years and 54 days. He said the secret to his longevity was being a healthy, small eater. In his words "Eat light to live long".

The title of the oldest person alive also belongs to a Japanese, Kane Tanaka. She was born on 2 January 1903, and she completes 117 years in 2020.

However, a Brazilian woman claims the title actually belongs to her. She was born on December 20 of 1900 and completed 119 years. Her family asked Guinness to give her the title. Her name is Maria Pereira dos Santos, she had 7 children, 16 grandsons, 24 great-grandsons, and 3 great-great-grandsons. She worked on a farm and lived a simple life. Unfortunately, she died in May of 2020, before completing 120 years.

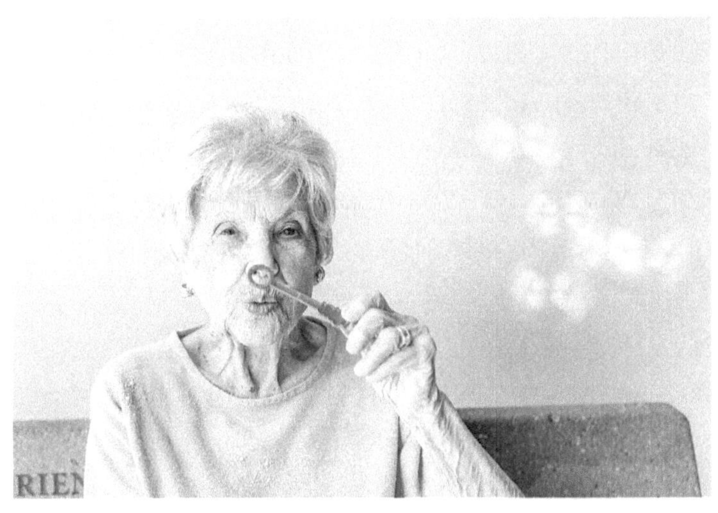

Is it possible to live for more than 120 years?

Anyway, she couldn´t beat the oldest person ever. This title belongs to Jeanne Louise Calment, a French woman who lived 122 years and 164 days. She was born on 21 February 1875, around 14 years before the Eiffel Tower was constructed (she saw it being built), and 15 years before the advent of movies. The year after her birth, Alexander Graham Bell patented the telephone.

She was rich so she never had to work, and she was engaged in various physical activities such as swimming, playing tennis, and cycling. He followed a healthy, rich in olive oil (which she also rubbed into her skin), and she liked to drink a glass of wine every now and then, no more than once per day. But she also had a sweet tooth, with a particular fondness for chocolate: she ate almost 1 kg (2 lb 3 oz) of it each week. Surprisingly, Jeanne had smoked almost her entire life.

She had a tranquil state of mind and a wonderful sense of humor. On her 120th birthday, journalists asked her what kind of future she expected. "A very short one," she replied.

As we saw, living 120, or even more, is possible. But what´s in common between these people? This is a question that intrigues scientists, and those who want to live longer and better lives.

Aging

Aging is defined as a gradual physiological deterioration that all living organisms experience with time. It´s a complex process that involves the accumulation of molecular and cellular damage leading to the decline of cells, affecting tissues and organs. The consequence is an increase in the susceptibility to diseases, and finally, death.

Healthy aging and longevity depend on a great variety of factors. Biologically speaking, this includes the integrity of the genetic material, regulation in protein function and homeostasis, and the length of the telomeres (the protective cap of our chromosomes). To live the longest we can, we must overcome the cellular and molecular decline that naturally occur as we age.

For our bodies to function properly, we need efficient communication between our cells.

Besides, our tissues and cells need to be regenerated once they´re damaged and substituted for new cells that can play their role.

There´s no single cause for the aging process. That´s why it ´s difficult to find a 'cure' for it. It involves genetic and environmental factors that are not yet fully elucidated (see review, Carmona and Michan, 2016).

• •

Calorie restriction – eating less to live longer

Jiroemon Kimura, a man who lived 116 years once said "Eat light to live long". Was he right?

Calorie restriction has been appointed as a robust method to increase longevity and delay aging and disease in various organisms. In experiments performed with lab rats, animals that were fed with 30 % less food lived 30 % longer than the ones that received regular chow diet (McKay and Maynard, 1935). This can be observed in other species too, such as yeast and monkeys.

In animal models, calorie restriction is capable of reducing the physiological biomarkers of aging such as osteoporosis, sarcopenia (loss of muscular force), body fat accumulation, and high blood sugar.

In humans, the effects of calorie restriction on longevity are not completely understood. We´ve had some examples trough history of involuntary calorie restriction.

This happened during World Wars I and II when local governments enforced food restriction with adequate consumption of nutritional-dense foods. During World War II, people in Norway were forced to reduce their calorie intake by 20 % for 4 years. Their diets were composed of fresh vegetables, potatoes, fish, and whole cereals. This measure decreased mortality by 30 % in both men and women (Strom and Jensen, 1951).

• •

Calorie restriction – eating less to live longer

Another example is the population of a Japanese island, Okinawa. This island has a huge number of centenarians (4 times higher than in other industrialized countries). They also have a decreased number of cases of cancer and heart diseases.

When scientists analyzed their diets, they noticed that adults living in Okinawa consumed approximately 17 % fewer calories than the average Japanese adult and 40 % fewer calories than an American adult. Their diet is also lower in protein, and rich in fresh vegetables and fruits, soy, and fish (Willcox et al., 2006). Nowadays, with the arrival of fast-food chains, the life expectancy for newborns in Okinawa is no longer different than in Japan.

A Randomized controlled study involving 220 healthy participants showed that 2 years of 25 % calorie restriction in humans can decrease fast insulin concentration and improve insulin sensitivity. The risk for cardiovascular diseases decreases by 29%. We can also observe a decline in oxidative stress, deposition of fat in the liver, and risk for type 2 diabetes (see review, Most et al., 2017).

In another study, body weight, insulin resistance, total cholesterol, LDL-cholesterol, triglycerides, and blood pressure decreased significantly and HDL-cholesterol increased in the 2 years of 25% calorie restriction group (see review, Most et al., 2017).

• •

Calorie restriction – eating less to live longer

As we have shown here, moderate calorie restriction can be beneficial in promoting healthy aging and preventing age-related diseases. More severe calorie restriction may be difficult to sustain in human beings, and it can cause side effects such as extreme leanness, loss of sex drive, cold sensitivity, and impairment in the menstrual cycle.

It´s important to notice that calorie restriction is only beneficial when the diet is composed of nutritional-rich food. Always consult with a doctor and a dietician to evaluate your nutritional needs.

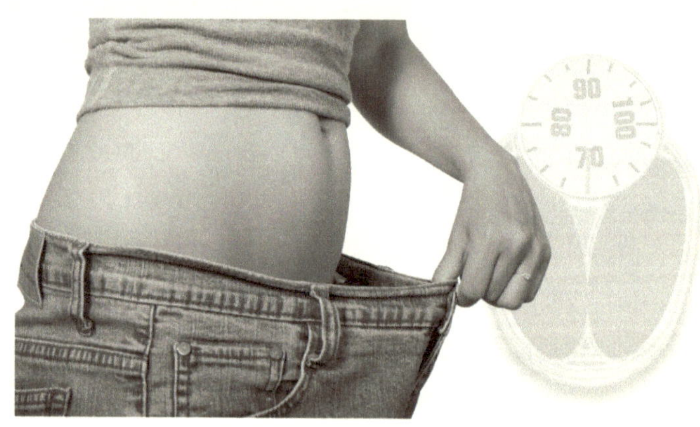

What can you eat to live longer?

By the year 2050, the global population of people with more than 60 years will double, achieving 2 billion, or 21 % of the World population. Besides, people are living longer. At the same time, there´s a concern for the health and quality of life of these people.

The consequences of unhealthy aging such as chronic age-related diseases can be prevented with lifestyle modification, including diet and exercise.

Healthy aging is not only living longer, it´s extending healthy active life. One way of doing this is by eliminating the major risk factors for chronic diseases such as smoking, lack of exercise, and a poor diet.

According to the World Health Organization (WHO), these measures can decrease up to 80 % of the risk for cardiovascular diseases, stroke, and type 2 diabetes.

As we age, we may not meet our nutritional requirements properly at the time we need it the most. This malnourishment is observed even in obese elderly people. This can happen due to several factors such as loss of appetite, changes in smell and taste, dental and chewing problems, limitations in mobility, and access to quality fresh food.

What can you eat to live longer?

Moreover, changes in the way food are absorbed in the stomach due to natural aging or to the use of certain medicines means that we may need more nutrients as we grow older. Besides, older adults tend to have an inadequate consumption of protein, fiber, vitamins, calcium, magnesium, and potassium. Older adults tend to report inadequate intakes of fruit, vegetables, legumes, whole grains, nuts or seeds, fish, lean meat, poultry, and low-fat fluid dairy products but excess intakes of refined grain products, processed and fatty meats, fried foods, solid fats, and added sugars.

Although supplements may be an option in the case of nutrients deficiency, they may not be more efficient than the whole food.

In general, high consumption of fruits and vegetables, whole grains, nuts, legumes, seeds, and low-fat dairy, moderate amounts of lean meat and fish, and limited consumption of refined/sugary foods can have a protective effect against cardiovascular diseases that are associated with the aging process.

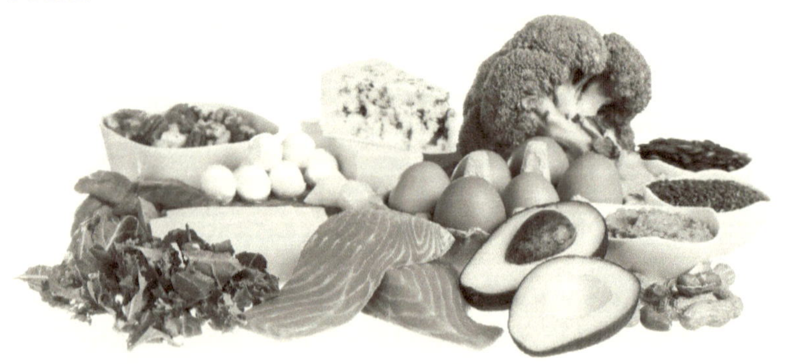

Omega-3 fatty acids are also important for the health of the cardiovascular system. In fact, low blood levels of omega-3 are found in people with coronary heart disease.

Research shows that it´s not the levels of omega-3 itself that are important, but the ratio between omega-3 and omega-6 fatty acids.

When the n-6: n-3 ratio decreases, telomere length increases. Long telomeres are associated with longer life. That´s because they protect our genetic material from damage.

Probably, individuals with higher endogenous n-6: n-3 polyunsaturated fatty acid ratios would have greater benefits from simple nutritional intervention in the form of omega-3 supplementation.

Consumption of vegetables, fruits, seeds, nuts, legumes, seaweeds, coffee, cereals, and whole grains was associated with longer telomeres (see review, Vidaček et al., 2016).

In summary, to healthier aging, you should limit the intake of energy-dense food while maximizing the intake of nutrient-rich food. A balanced diet is key to healthy aging and better quality of life.

As we said before, it´s important to consult a dietician to make a correct evaluation of your nutritional needs.

Physical activity

The health benefits of physical activity are already well known. Exercising can do wonderful things for the health of your body and mind. But can exercising help you live longer? We already know that exercising reduces the risk of developing cardiovascular disease and diabetes by maintaining control of the levels of cholesterol, triglycerides, and sugar in the blood. Physical activity also improves blood circulation, maintains healthy arterial pressure, and strengthens the immune system. This means that you are better protected against diseases and infections.

Another positive outcome of physical activity in older people is that it helps developing balance and it reduces the risk of falls, thus reducing mortality.

It´s also important in helping building muscles since older people experience muscular loss.

Overall, a healthy lifestyle not only decreases the risk of diseases but also slows down disease progression such as cancer, for example.

Additionally, physical activity was positively correlated with great telomere length, and sedentary behavior was associated with shorter telomeres in research studies.

This is an area that needs further investigation because we don´t know yet the depth of this relationship (see review, Vidaček et al., 2016).

Physical activity

A minimum of 150 minutes per week of moderate physical activity is recommended to maintain a healthy body (WHO). People who adhere to this recommendation have 26 % lower chances of developing type 2 diabetes than sedentary people.

Age is the greatest risk factor for developing cancer. Over 60% of people who have cancer are older than 65. Exercise may also have a role in cancer prevention. In fact, physical activity is associated with a decreased risk of 13 cancers both for individuals who are overweight/obese and normal-weight.

Moreover, people who are physically active after a diagnosis of cancer such as breast cancer or colorectal have higher chances of survival than those who don´t exercise (see review, Pedersen, 2019).

Dementia is a syndrome associated with a decline in brain functioning that involves memory loss, difficulties in speaking, mood changes, and other symptoms. One example of dementia is Alzheimer's disease. One in 14 people over 65 develops dementia.

Studies suggest that regular exercise decreases the risk of Alzheimer´s by 40% (see review, Pedersen, 2019).

That said, physical exercise can prevent most diseases associated with aging and promote healthy aging, thereby increasing life span and healthy active life.

• •

• •

Stress

Stress is one of the mechanisms that are closely related to the aging process. Resisting this stress is a way to prevent the occurrence of age-related diseases, thus slowing aging itself.

But at least for now, we´re not talking about psychological stress. Other types of stressors can affect our body, such as oxidative stress, inflammation, thermal stress, heavy metals, and UV-light exposure. Scientists believe that if your body can resist well to all of these different stressors, it´ll resist the aging process as well.

As an example, fruit-flies and worms that carry a mutation (a modification into their genetic code) which increases their lifespan also confer resistance to multiple-stressors. Besides, animals that naturally live longer demonstrate forms of stress resistance.

But what´s the relevance of this for humans? It´s possible that learning how to increase our body´s resistance to stress can help us find a way to increase our lifespan.

Calorie restriction for example is long-term energetic stress that results in increased lifespan. Moreover, periodic fasting is known to reduce the risk of age-related diseases such as diabetes and cardiovascular diseases.

Other transient stressors were tested, such as heat and cold stress. However, the results of these experiments are still inconclusive.

• •

Oxidative stress

We can define oxidative stress as the imbalance between the production of highly oxidative compounds and the antioxidant defense of our body, leading to tissue damage.

The oxygen metabolism generates lots of free radicals and non-radical reactive oxygen species (ROS). The antioxidant system offers protection against this free-radicals, reducing the damage caused by them to our cells and tissues.

Some scientists believe that the accumulation of oxidative damage to our molecules can lead to the functional decline that happens as we age.

Oxidative stress plays an important role in aging. This is because the increase in the ROS levels leads to cellular senescence, meaning that cells stop proliferating due to damage that occurs during their replication. These cells start to secrete molecules involved in the immune response such as interleukins, chemokines, growth factors, and degradative enzymes.

This process is involved in the development of age-related diseases such as cardiovascular diseases, kidney diseases, neurodegenerative diseases, and cancer.

• •

Oxidative stress

That´s why scientists created a theory to explain the aging process. According to this theory, aging is a loss of homeostasis due to chronic oxidative stress that affects especially the nervous, endocrine, and immune systems. The activation of the immune system leads to an inflammatory state that creates a vicious circle in which chronic oxidative stress and inflammation feed each other, thus increasing the age-related morbidity and mortality (see review, Liguori et al., 2018).

How to overcome this?

To prevent oxidative stress from happening, our body needs anti-oxidants. Well-known antioxidants are vitamins A, C, and E. Consuming the right amount of each of these vitamins decreases the risk of developing age-related diseases. However, it´s not clear if they impact mortality, or if they can be used as an anti-oxidant therapy.

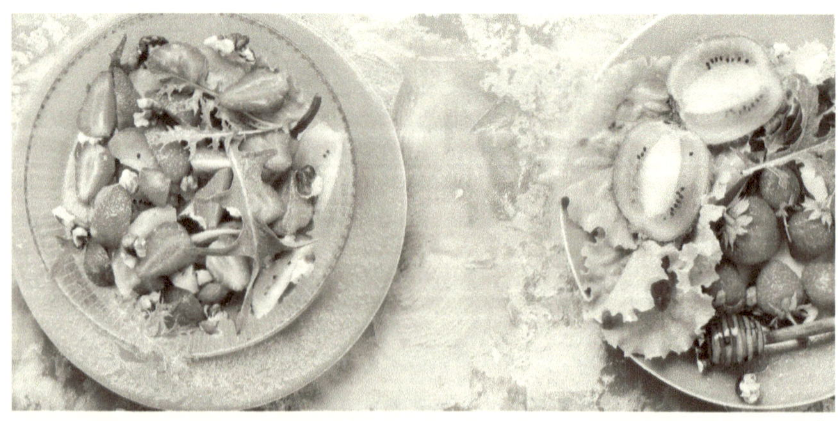

• •

Vitamins

- **Vitamin A** – also known as retinol, it´s found in eggs, cheese, oily fish, milk, and liver. You can get vitamin A by consuming yellow food containing beta-carotene such as carrots and mango. Vitamin A participates in the body´s defense against infection, and in maintaining your skin and vision healthy.
- **Vitamin C** – also known as ascorbic acid, it´s found in orange, strawberries, and broccoli. Vitamin C is important in wound healing and it maintains the health of the skin, bones, and cartilage.
- **Vitamin E** – it´s found in plant oils, nuts, seeds, and cereals. It helps to maintain the health of the skin and eyes, and it strengthens the body´s natural defense against illness.

Remember: Too much vitamin can be useless, or even harmful. It´s important to stick to the ideal daily intake of each vitamin. The best way to achieve this is through a balanced diet.

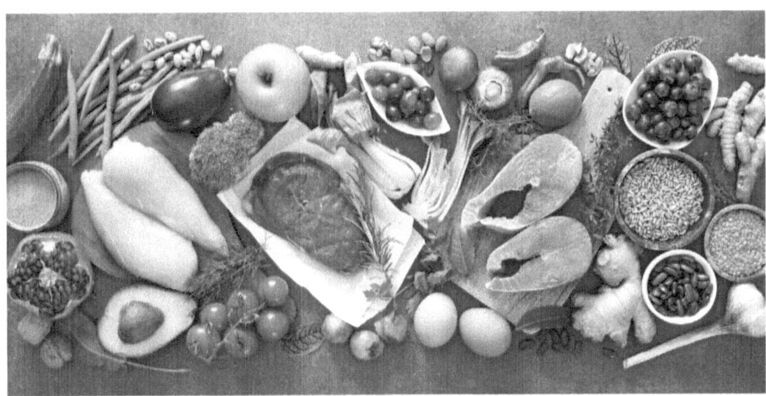

Polyphenols – drink wine and eat chocolate to live longer

Polyphenols are found in fruits, vegetables, cereals, and beverages. A glass of wine contains 100 mg of polyphenols. They can be divided into flavonoids and non-flavonoids.

One example of flavonoid is quercetin, it´s present in wine, and it can prevent the occurrence of cardiovascular diseases and cancer. It also has an anti-inflammatory effect.

Resveratrol is an example of a non-flavonoid, also found in wine. Resveratrol may explain a thing called the "French-paradox". This is because French people have a low incidence of cardiovascular diseases besides their high consumption of saturated fat. They consume 20-30 g of wine per day.

This substance can bring health benefits such as reducing vascular inflammation, preventing hypertension, reducing LDL cholesterol, increasing HDL cholesterol, and improving insulin sensitivity, thus preventing diabetes. All of these factors are associated with decreased risk of cardiovascular diseases.

Resveratrol can also help to prevent neurodegenerative diseases, cancer, and osteoporosis.

We can also find resveratrol in dark chocolate, grapes, berries, and peanuts. Maybe this was Jeanne Louise Calment ´s big secret, who knows?

• • • • • • • • • • • • •

• •

Psychological stress

More than live longer, we want to live better. There´s no point in reaching longevity without a healthy mind.
We know that with age, the risk of developing mental health issues increases. Like the other stressors we discussed here, psychological stress also has a role in the aging process. According to WHO, there´s a proportional increase in projected lifetime risk versus prevalence of mood disorders. This means that the more stressed a person is, the more chances of developing mood disorders, which will have a negative clinical effect by accelerating aging, and mortality. Thus, people that are more resilient to stress will probably have less age-related mood disorders, and consequently, will live a longer and better life.
Resilience is the capacity of recovering quickly from difficulties. When we face a stressful situation, our body responds by activating the HPA (hypothalamic-pituitary-adrenal) axis. The HPA axis is a neuroendocrine system that plays an important role in the stress response. It releases cortisol, the stress hormone.
Prolonged exposition to the stressor can lead to chronic stress. The consequences will depend on the ability of each person to adapt to it. Sometimes, the stress response is exacerbated, the individual can´t recover properly and develop a susceptibility to stress.

• •

Psychological stress

Others are less vulnerable, or resilient. Less resilient people tend to develop a mental illness such as anxiety and depression more easily.

This vulnerability depends on several factors, such as genetic predisposition, social and environmental factors, the presence of chronic illness, and the exposure to stress early in life.

Stress resilience becomes even more important as we age and it's a critical factor in maintaining health and longevity. A research group studied centenarians, nonagenarians, and octogenarians, and found that nonagenarians aged 94-98 with increased resilience had a 43.1% higher likelihood of living to be 100 or becoming a centenarian than those with lower resilience.

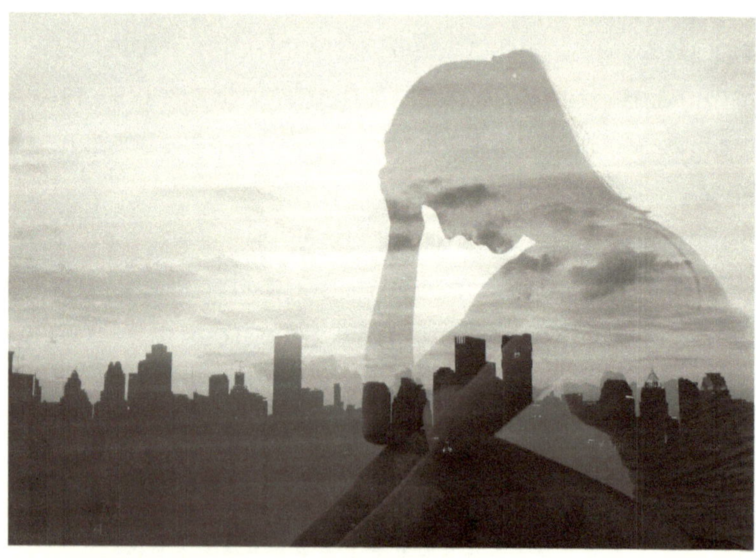

How to build stress resilience?

Behavioral approaches to build stress resilience are based on targeting positive emotions, problem-solving, life purpose, and cognitive flexibility.

Regular exercise is another way to improve general well-being and lowering the risk for mood disorders, probably enhancing resilience to stress. In fact, people who exercise regularly are more resistant to the emotional effects of acute stress and this might protect them against diseases related to chronic stress burden (see review, Faye et al., 2018).

The reasons why an older person loses resilience and how to get it back are areas of research that need to be further explored.

Building resilience is like building a muscle, it requires training and effort. Here you can see some tips from the American Psychological Association (APA) to overcome bad experiences and grow from the difficulties.

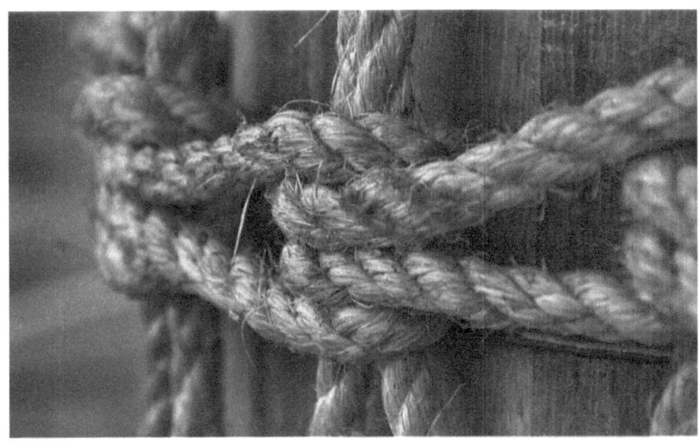

How to build stress resilience?

- **Prioritize your relationships**: remember you´re not alone in difficult times, surround yourself from supportive, empathetic, and trustworthy people. Don´t isolate yourself, try to connect with the ones who care for you. You may consider joining a group, for example.
- **Take care of your body**: proper nutrition, hydration, sleep, and regular exercise can make wonderful things for your mental health, and it can help your body to adapt to stress and reduce depression and anxiety.
- **Find purpose**: you can do this by helping others, volunteering, or simply offering support for the people you know that are in need.
- **Be proactive**: ask yourself what you can do to solve your problem. If it seems too difficult, break in smaller pieces and try to manage them. Taking initiative will remind you of your motivation and purpose.
- **Have a goal in mind**: set realistic goals and celebrate every accomplishment, even the small ones.
- **Embrace positive thoughts**: seeing the glass half-full can help you expect that good things will happen to you. This will make it easier to achieve the things that you want and to act positively.

How to build stress resilience?

- **Keep things in perspective**: you may not be able to change a highly stressful event, but you can change how you interpret and respond to it.
- **Accept change**: change is part of life. Instead of focusing on things you can´t change, focus on circumstances that you can alter.
- **Seek help**: getting help when you need it is crucial in building your resilience. For this purpose, you can consult with a licensed mental health professional.

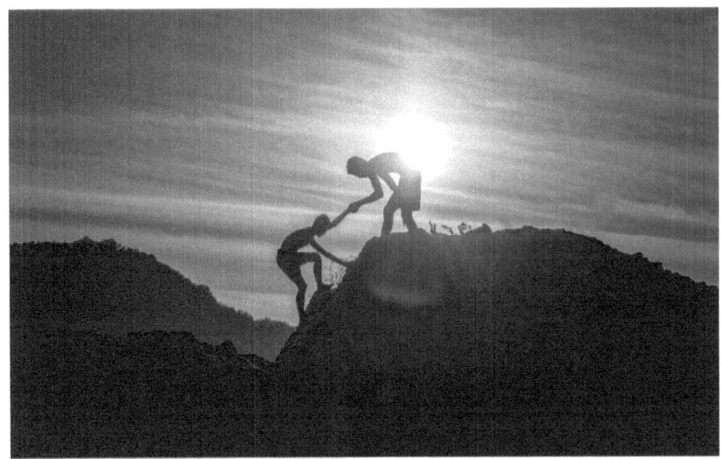

Meditation and Yoga

Meditation is another intervention that can be very helpful in reducing psychological stress.

Meditation is associated with lower levels of anxiety, and depression, as well as higher levels of self-esteem and satisfaction.

People who meditate regularly show increased attention and greater capacity for introspection, self-awareness, self-control, and management of emotions.

Meditation teaches us to observe and more fully enjoy the experiences that life offers, enhancing our emotional and intuitive intelligence.

One research was carried out with 35 men with prostate cancer. One group practiced yoga and meditation as part of a lifestyle change program. Compared to the control group, they had an increase in 10 % in the length of the telomeres. Similarly, telomeres shortening after radiotherapy was smaller in women who practiced yoga. The same result can be observed regarding mindfulness meditation.

Somewhat, both meditation and yoga seem to confer a protective effect over our DNA, preventing age-associated damage and oxidative stress (see review, Mrithunjay, and Abraham, 2018).

Meditation and Yoga

Yoga can bring several health benefits such as reducing arterial pressure, decreasing the levels of LDL cholesterol, and increasing the levels of HDL cholesterol. Blood sugar control is also improved.

An extra benefit of yoga on healthy aging is that it improves balance, physical fitness, and flexibility, reducing the risk of falls in older people. It also promotes greater cognitive functioning, and overall well-being (see review, Field, 2016).

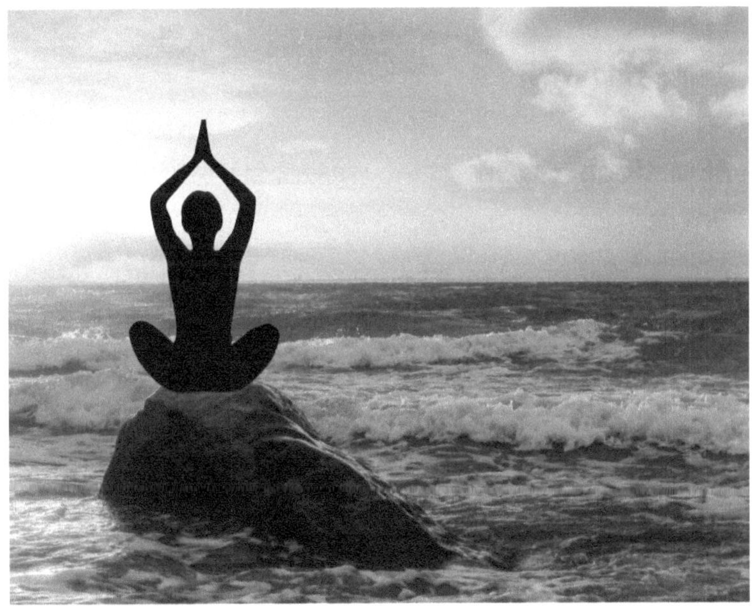

Sleep more to live more

Sleep is a fundamental behavior characterized by reduced responsiveness to sensory stimuli and suppressed locomotor activity, which can be quickly reversed to wakefulness. We can divide human sleep into 4 stages:

- **Non-REM sleep**: in this stage, you´ll progressively lose your consciousness. Non-REM sleep is divided into three stages:
    - N1
    - N2
    - N3 – also known as the deepest sleep, or slow-wave sleep (SWS).

- **REM sleep** (rapid eye movement sleep): this is the stage where spontaneous rapid eye movements occur. You won´t be able to move (muscular atonia), and it´ll be more difficult to wake you under stimuli. This is also the stage where you dream.

In a regular night of sleep, you´ll alternate between these different stages, including non-REM (N1, N2, N3) and REM sleep.

Consequences of sleep loss

Due to our daily obligations with work, study, family, house chores, and social life, we live in a world where sleep seems like the least important thing. But the truth is you´re probably sleeping less than your body needs. This is known as sleep restriction, one of the reasons sleep problems are skyrocketing in our society. With this negligence, comes the consequences.

Regularly restricting your sleep can lead to chronic sleep loss, which can affect your health. Some of the negative consequences can be:

- **Weight gain**: when you don´t get enough sleep you feel hungrier and less satisfied. It´s more likely you´ll crave sweets, salty and starchy food, which can potentially make you gain some extra weight.

- **Immune system impairment**: when sleep-deprived, you´ll catch a cold easier, and your body won´t recover quickly from infections as well.

- **Mood disorders**: when sleep-restricted, you tend to feel more irritated, anxious, and depressed. Your memory is also affected.

- **Cardiovascular diseases**: sleep loss increases blood pressure and the risk of developing cardiovascular diseases.

Consequences of sleep loss

- **Safety issues**: a bad night of sleep can make it hard to concentrate on everyday tasks. That´s why driving or operating heavy machines can be dangerous and not recommended.
- **Productivity**: sleeping less than you need may impair your productivity levels, since you may feel moody and have daytime fatigue. Your concentration is affected as well, which may have a huge impact on your productivity at difficult tasks.
- **Mortality**: sleeping less than 6 hours a night is associated with increased all-cause mortality. According to the National Sleep Foundation, an adult should sleep 7 – 9 hours a night.

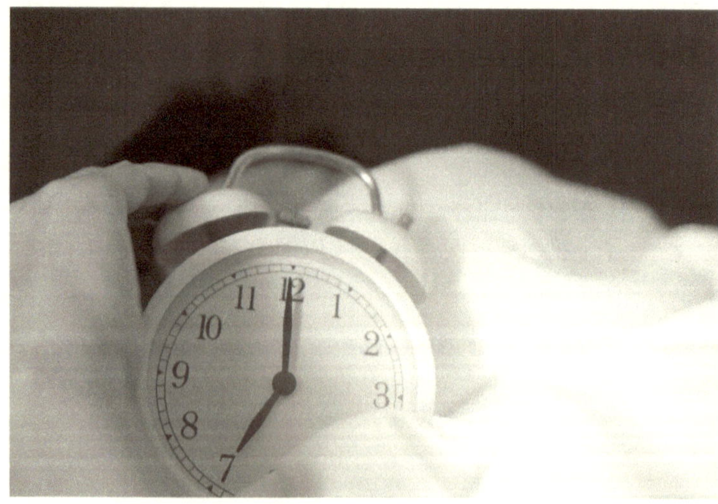

Sleep and aging

Sleep patterns change during our life. Babies have polyphasic sleep, which means that they sleep and wake up several times during the day. With time, they begin to establish their sleep at night but continue to do a few naps during the day. Teens tend to go to bed later and wake up later than adults. Adults usually sleep between 7 and 8 hours at night. Some people like to do a nap after lunch.

If you're older than 60 years, of life with someone who is, you might have noticed that sleep is not the same when compared to a younger person. This is perfectly natural since some changes in the sleep pattern occur as we age. Older people tend to go to bed earlier and to wake up earlier than younger adults.

Older adults also experience more difficulty falling asleep, shorter sleep duration, and sleep fragmentation, meaning they wake up several times during the night.

Besides, they spend more time in the lighter phases of sleep and their sleep is more fragile, meaning it´s easier for them to wake up. Of course, not all people will experience the same changes in the same degrees.

Sleep and aging

Sleep disruption is also observed in neurodegenerative diseases. In fact, they can seem years before the onset of the disease. Poor quality sleep may facilitate the development of dementia. Moreover, sleep disturbances such as insomnia and sleep apnea increase the risk of dementia.

This suggests that inadequate sleep is not only a predisposing risk factor contributing to neurodegenerative disease, but represents a novel treatment opportunity and/or even preventative strategy in this context.

That being said, to live a longer and better life, sleep should be one of your top priorities. That´s because poor quality sleep and insufficient sleep is associated with a variety of age-related diseases.

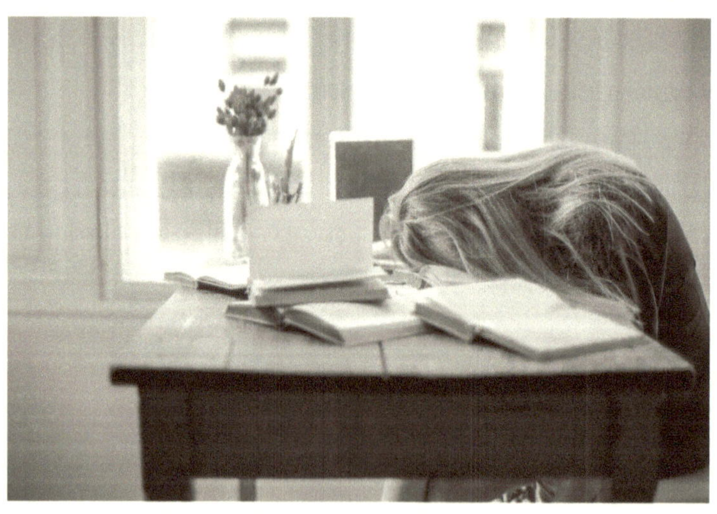

Tips for better sleep quality

If you want to have a better sleep quality, you can follow these simple steps also known as sleep hygiene.

- **Exercise during the day**: exercise can have a huge impact on your sleep quality. It´s best to avoid extensive workouts close to bedtime. However, the effect of intense nighttime exercise on sleep differs from person to person, so try to find out what works best for you.
- **Avoid long naps during the day**: naps longer than 30 minutes may spoil your nighttime sleep.
- **Make sure that your sleep environment is pleasant:** sleep has to be a pleasant experience for you. Everything in the environment must be cozy and comfortable, from mattresses and pillows to the room itself. It´s important to turn off all the lights, including the TV, computer and cellphone. You can use blackout curtains, eyeshades, earplugs, "white noise" machines, humidifiers, and other devices that can make the bedroom feel more relaxing for you.
- **Avoid stimulants such as alcohol or caffeine near bedtime:** coffee can make you feel awake and agitated during the night. Drinking alcohol near bedtime can disrupt your sleep, and you´ll wake up feeling terrible.

Tips for better sleep quality

- **Have a regular sleep-waking schedule**: our bodies function like clocks. A regular schedule for eating, exercising, and sleeping will help your internal clock to synchronize to the external environment. A regular nightly routine helps your body recognize that it is bedtime. So naturally, you´ll feel sleepy at night, and awake when the sun rises.
- **Expose yourself to daylight early in the morning**: this will help your internal clock synchronize to the external light/dark cycle, and your brain and body will understand when it´s time for sleep, and wake up.
- **Avoid light exposure during the night** (avoid computer and cellphone near bedtime). Blue light in these devices interferes with the production of melatonin (sleep inductor hormone), interfering with your sleep quality.
- **Only go to bed when you´re sleepy**: if you use your bed for other purposes, such as eating, reading, and working, your brain will get confused. If you go to bed only when it's time for sleep, your brain will understand that it´s bedtime.
- **Avoid stressful situations near bedtime**: stress makes you release a hormone called cortisol, which will keep you awake.

Tips for better sleep quality

- **Have a healthy diet and avoid fatty, fried, heavy food near bedtime:** these types of food can trigger indigestion for some people. When this occurs close to bedtime, it can lead to painful heartburn that disrupts sleep.

These tips can be followed by people of any age. If you´re experiencing sleep problems, seek specialized help.

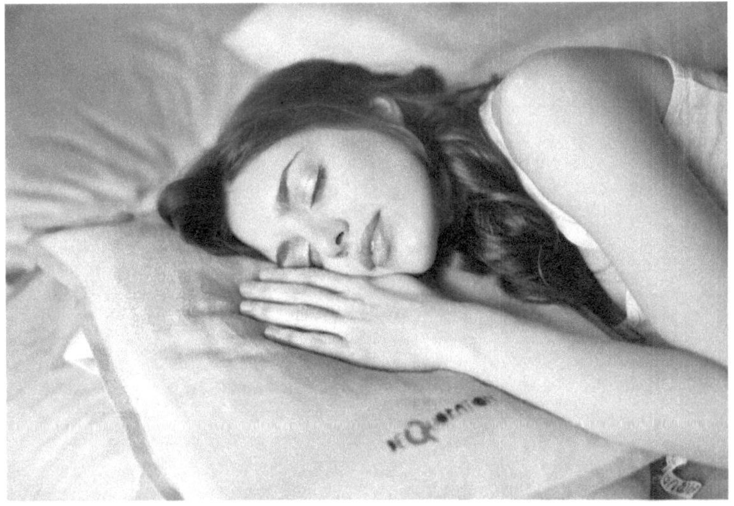

What makes us live longer?

Life expectancy is a metric that directly reflects how healthy people are. In the pre-modern world, you´d be considered an elder if you made it past 30.
Fortunately for those who live in the 21st century, things have changed considerably since then. We can thank industrialization for that. In the early 19th century, life expectancy started to increase in industrialized countries, while it remained low in the rest of the world.
The consequences of this inequality can be seen today. The poorest countries, which took longer to develop, still face major public health problems and a shorter life expectancy when compared to the wealthier countries. For example, in 2019 the country with the lowest life expectancy is the Central African Republic with 53 years, in Japan life expectancy is 30 years longer (Roser et al., 2013).
On the map below, you can find information about life expectancy across the world. In countries where public health is poor, life expectancy does not exceed 60 years.

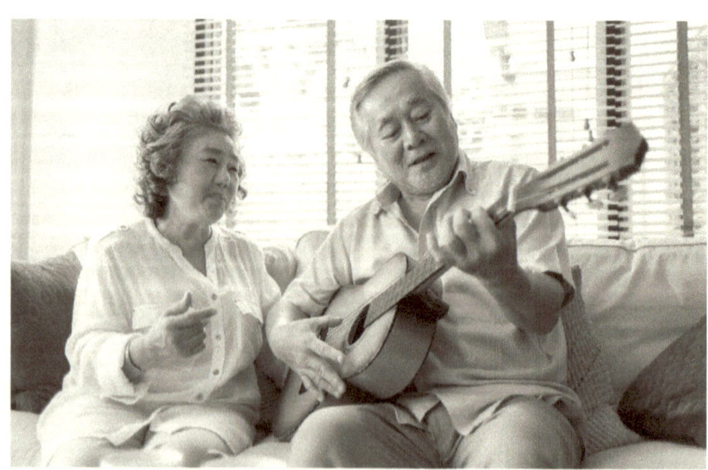

What makes us live longer?

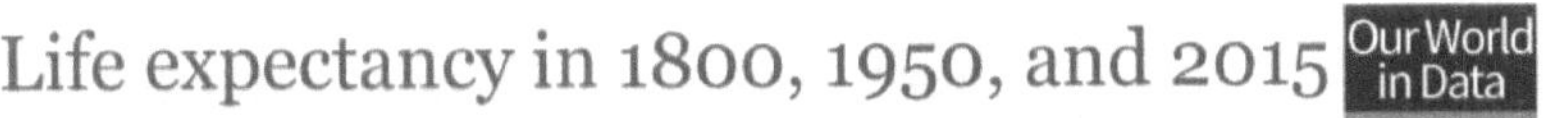

Life expectancy in 1800, 1950, and 2015

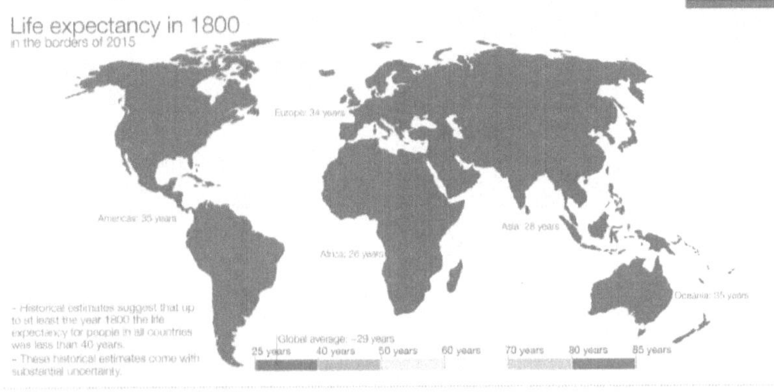

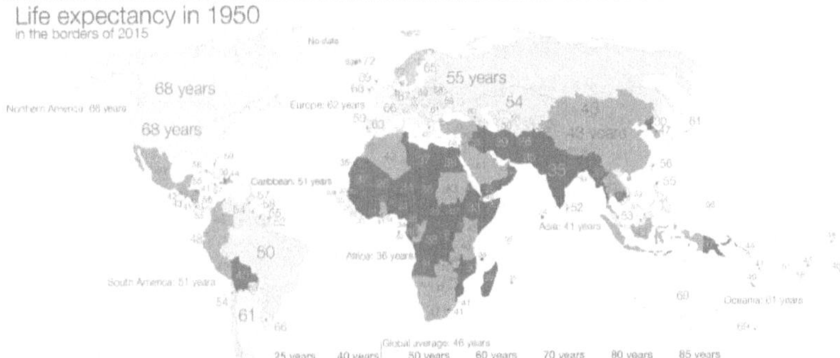

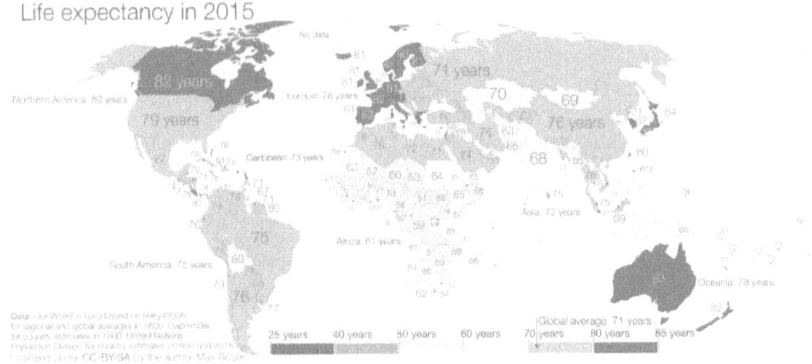

35

Life expectancy has changed over the years

In the 19th century, people lived no longer than 40.
At that time, we had little knowledge about medicine and hygiene was also very poor.
The lack of basic sanitation and simple hygiene habits were a great opportunity for viruses and bacteria to proliferate and cause disease. Also, those who were injured in wars or even at work were vulnerable to infections. Believe it or not, doctors only started to wash their hands before surgery after 1867. This year, Dr. Joseph Lister published an article showing how to clean wounds, killing the germs, and preventing infection (Lister, 1867).
Another event that has changed the course of medicine was the discovery of penicillin by Alexander in 1928. However, it´s clinical use was only possible 10 years later (Gaynes, 2017). This means that it has been only 79 years since we first had an effective treatment for bacterial infections.
In 1950 life expectancy was already 60 years in Europe, North America, Oceania, Japan and parts of South America. Global inequality remained huge, while in Norway people were expected to live until 72 years, in Mali they lived 26 years on average (Roser et al., 2013).
Since then, all regions in the world have made substantial progress. Globally the life expectancy increased from 30 to 72 years in 2019 (United Nations Department for Economic and Social Affairs, 2019).

Life expectancy has changed over the years

And we won´t stop there just yet. By 2040, all countries are expected to see an increase in lifespan. One study estimated that global life expectancy will increase by 4.4 years. This is because over 36 diseases are expected to decline or disappear (Foreman et al., 2018).

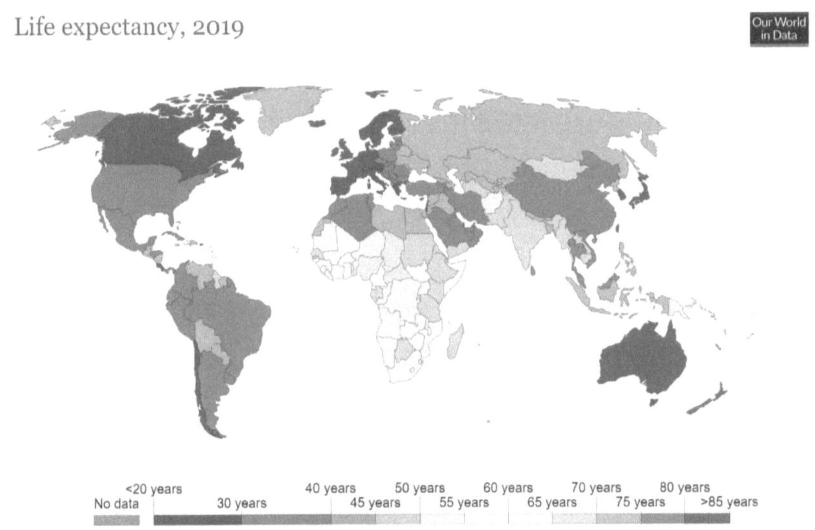

With the majority of people reaching a certain age, we expect to see some points out of the curve. Will the number with more than 100 years increase in the next few decades? This trend is already proving to be true. In the United Kingdom (UK), there were half a million people aged 90 or more in 2015. Between 2005 and 2015, the number of centenarians increased by 65%, and the number of people with more than 105 doubled in the same period. Although women tend to live longer, we are seeing an increase in men´s lifespan. It is expected that in 2043, 20.8% of newborn boys and 26.1% of newborn girls will live to at least 100 years of age (Office for National Statistics, 2016).

Things won´t be different in the U.S. By 2060, American's life expectancy is projected to increase by 6 years (from 79.9 in 2017 to 85.6 in 2060). By 2034 the population over 65 will outline the population under age 18 for the first time in history (Medina et al., 2020).

In 2016 there were 82,000 centenarians in the U.S and this number is expected to increase to 589,000 by 2060 (U.S. Census Bureau).

The other side of the coin

Advances in medicine, such as the discovery of antibiotics and vaccines, in addition to better living conditions with more people with access to drinking water and basic sanitation, have made the world population leap in the last century. People are taking better care of themselves, thanks to the success of health prevention programs, which has also contributed to the increase in life expectancy, especially in more developed countries.

However, the aging of the population has its consequences, which makes it important that countries plan public policies to guarantee dignified and healthy aging for their inhabitants. The first thing we have to consider is that living longer does not necessarily mean living healthier.

There are a great number of diseases that are associated with aging such as diabetes, hypertension, cardiovascular diseases, dementia, disability, depression, cancer, and so on. In the U.S., severe disability fell 25% from 1982 to 2001, which could be a positive indication of how we will function as we age. However, the rise in obesity may negatively impact these numbers.

The other side of the coin

One report showed that American adults have worse health when compared to Europeans, regardless of income. This was due to the presence of chronic diseases and measures of disability. Cognitive functioning declined further between ages 55 and 65 in countries where workers left the labor force at an early age, suggesting that engagement in work might help preserve cognitive functioning (Avendano et al., 2009).

Having more older people in the population will have implications for public health, social services, and health care systems. Public expenses with health will likely increase considerably.

The WHO Study on Global Ageing and Adult Health (SAGE) aims to investigate people over 50 years of age from 6 different countries (China, Ghana, India, Mexico, Russia, and South Africa). Preliminary data of this research showed that age is associated with an increase in blood pressure among women.

Since hypertension is linked to cerebrovascular and cardiac diseases that are likely to require expensive medical treatments. That´s why it is important to invest in early detection and on effective management of the risk factors. This could potentially reduce the burden of age-related chronic diseases.

The other side of the coin

After cardiac disease, cancer is the second cause of death in the U.S. The financial costs of cancer are high for both the patient and society. It was estimated that the direct medical costs for cancer in the U.S. in 2015 were $80.2 billion (The Agency for Healthcare Research and Quality - AHRQ). Because of aging, the incidence of cancer is expected to increase. The annual number of new cancer cases is projected to rise to 17 million by 2020 and reach 27 million by 2030.

Therefore, governments (especially in developing countries) should invest in prevention and early diagnosis programs so that the disease is discovered in its early stages when the chances of a better prognosis are higher (NIH, 2011).

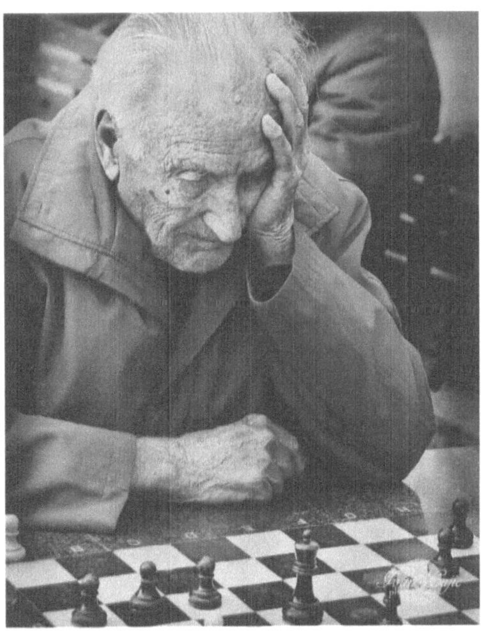

Work

In developed countries, older people live the workforce once they achieve a certain age. Some continue productive participating in the informal workforce, volunteering, or helping their families.

Retirement is based on age (or years of contribution) rather than on health-related problems. In the U.S people live an average of 20 years after retirement (USA.gov). Many countries now want people working for more years since the costs of pensions are escalating.

To maintain people with over 65 years of age working, we need to change some misconceptions. Many older people have intact cognitive functioning and are capable of contributing to a company due to their skills and knowledge. The permanence of older people in the workforce will depend on the jobs that are available to them.

Jobs which demand physical strength may not be the most suitable, for example.

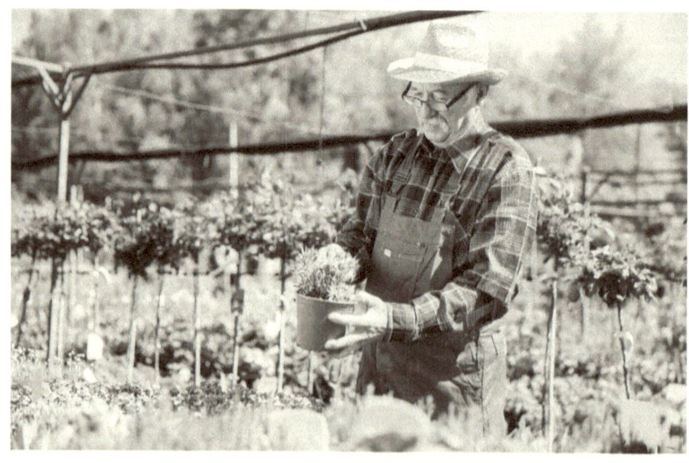

Family

With an aging population and increased longevity, more people will have the opportunity to meet their grandparents and great-grandparents. Today we have something that was not possible before, the coexistence between people of several generations in the same family.

However, people are choosing to have fewer children, or even not to have children at all. Besides, we have fewer people in the same family living together and there are family members who live in distant locations.

This could implicate less care and support for older people in the future. The percentage of older people living alone is increasing in most countries. In some European countries, more than 40% of women aged 65 or more live alone.

In the past, older people living alone was considered a signal of loneliness. However, this conception is changing. Many older people prefer to stay in their own homes as they age.

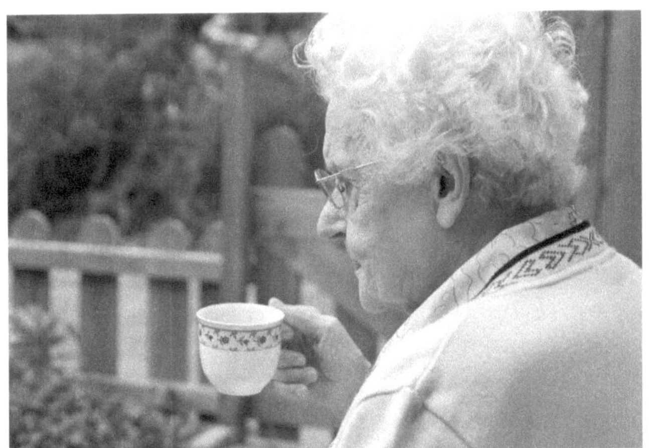

Long-term care

As people get older, some people may develop illnesses that cause disability or limit mobility. Therefore, they may need long-term care.

This care can be performed at home by a family member or caregiver, in a nursing home, or even in a hospital, which will generate costs for the family and society.

In less developed countries, it is common for a family member to have to leave school or work to care for an older relative.

This can be avoided if we find ways to reduce disability among older people. The big challenge will be to keep older people healthy for longer.

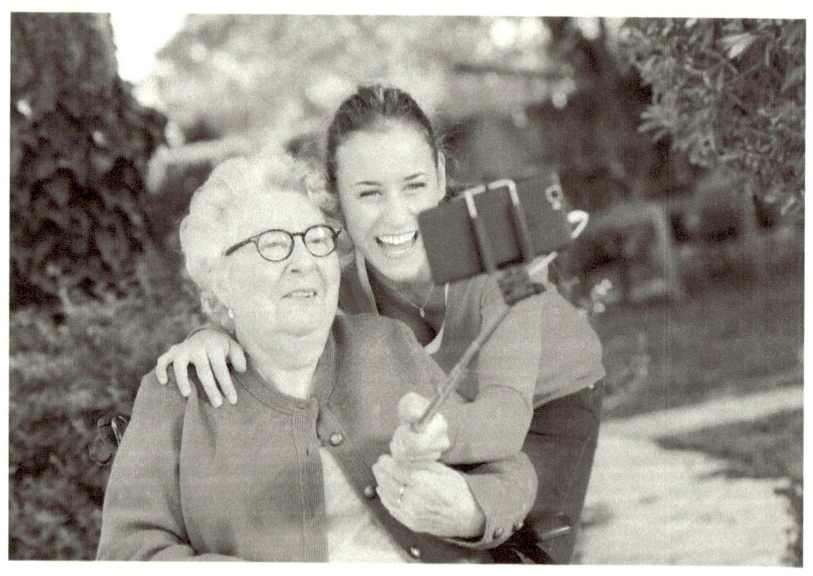

Aging in place

With the increase in the elderly population, it is essential to seek solutions so that these people can age with dignity and quality of life. One way to do that is to respect their decisions. "I want to stay in my own home" – This is what many older people say when asked about where they want to live as they age. 90% of people with over 65 want to age in place for as long as possible.

However, some of them can´t take care of themselves alone. They need support to perform daily activities such as taking a bath, preparing food, eating, cleaning the house, taking their medicines, and buying groceries.

How to respect their will and still provide the care they need?

Luckily, having all of the support without having to leave your home is possible. This is called aging in place which means staying in your own home as you get older. For some people, this could be choosing a retirement house that offers a home-like environment.

Nowadays, you can get almost all the support you need at home just by hiring a specialized service.

Aging in place

Examples of services available are:
- Personal care – older adults with movement limitations may need help to perform their hygiene. Having someone to help them with this is essential. It can be a relative or a caregiver.
- Household chores – cleaning the house and cooking may get difficult for older people. It´s important to have the support of a relative for this, or hiring a specialized service. Another option is to use food delivery apps or buying pre-prepared meals for the week.
- Money management – it may become difficult to manage so many bills and taxes. Try to organize your bills to pay them on time and avoid interests. You can ask someone of trust to do this for you. Try to use your bank´s app to pay most of the bills and put them on automatic debit, if possible.
- Health care – some people with age-related diseases may need specialized support which can be made at home with the help of a nurse, a physiotherapist, or a caregiver. They may also need help to take their medication on time.
- Social support – it´s very important to remain as social as you age. Stay in touch with your family and friends, visit them or let them visit when possible, and participate in your community´s groups and associations.

- Transportation – older adults with limited movement or disability may need help to go to appointments, shopping, or social activities. It´s important to have the support of a relative or else, to hire a specialized service. Apps can also be used, be sure to always share the information of the car and driver with someone you trust.

Aging in place can be very beneficial because it honors the choice and dignity of the older person, maintains familiarity and comfort, increases the quality of life, encourages independence, decreases depression and the feeling of loneliness and abandonment, reduces the risk of getting infectious diseases, and reduces the stress associated with living in a retirement home.

Aging in place needs to be planned if that´s your choice or the choice of someone in your family.

To begin with, you should consider what type of help you may need when you get older. If you live with other people, you should talk to them about your plans and the possibility of including them. If you live alone, you won´t have anyone to help you when necessary.

Aging in place

Pre-existing illnesses should be taken into account. Several age-related diseases can cause limitations. Therefore, it is a good idea to talk to your doctor about how these health problems can make it difficult for you or the person living with you to perform daily tasks.

Talk to your friends and relatives about the possibility of having someone to assist you. Finally, make your house accessible, especially if you have mobility problems. It´s best to make some changes to make your life easier and safer.

It's also very important to be financially prepared, especially if you can´t rely only on your relatives to assist you during this time. Some of the services will have a cost, others may be free, or covered by your health insurance. Being informed about the type of services and support that your country offers is also essential.

In the U.S. for example, there is a federal health insurance program for people 65 and older called Medicare. It´s not entirely free, but it´s cheaper than health insurance considering long-term care.

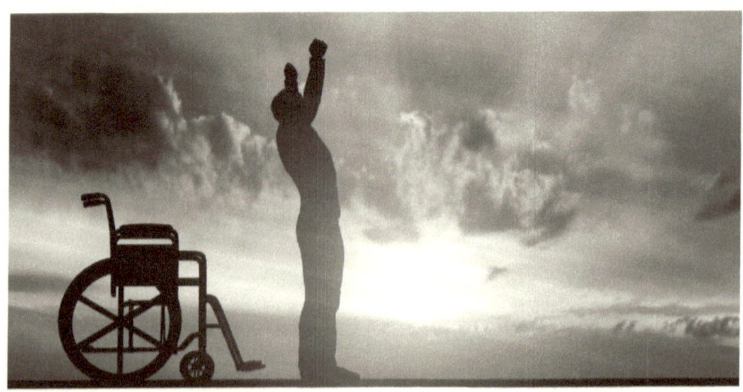

The secrets of the centenarians living in the "blue zones"

Blue zones are the regions on the planet where people live longer and better than the average.
According to Dan Buettner (2012), 5 blue zones exist in the world:

- Ikaria, Greece – this island near Turkey has one of the world´s lowest rates of middle-age mortality and dementia. The increased longevity of the population can be associated with the Mediterranean diet which is based on vegetables and healthy fats. They also consume less dairy and meat.
- ·Okinawa, Japan – this is the place with more centenarians in the world. Besides eating a healthy diet, older residents of Okinawa show very low levels of depression. They are very active and practice physical activity such as karate, dancing, walking, or riding a bike. The reduced stress can he attributed to tai-chi and meditation. They are social, and generally seek activities involving the community. Also, their positive attitude towards life helps to alleviate stress.
- Ogliastra, Sardinia – this Italian island has the greatest concentration of centenarian men. Their diet is low in protein, which is associated with lower rates of diabetes and cancer.

The secrets of the centenarians living in the "blue zones"

- Loma Linda, California – this region concentrates the biggest Adventists community in the U.S. Their diet is based on grains, fruits, nuts, and vegetables which is associated with an increase in longevity. The life expectancy of this population is 10 years greater than the average.
- Nicoya Peninsula, Costa Rica – this island in Central America has the lowest rate of middle-age mortality and the second biggest concentration of male centenarians. The residents of this island are social and practice regular low-intensity physical activity.

Is there a longevity gene?

The key to longevity is likely a combination of environment and genetics. One study done by the New England Centenarian Study at Boston University suggested that there is an association between human longevity and the HLA-DRB1 and/or HLA-DQ genes. This gene provides instructions for making a protein that plays a critical role in the immune system. More studies are needed to establish a link between longevity and genetics (Mishra, 2009).

● ●

Super centenarians are the Eyewitnesses to History

Most people learned history by reading a book, watching a documentary, or listening to a teacher. But there is nothing more valuable than learning by listening to people who have been there and experienced that moment.

Jerry Friedman, author of the book "Earth's Elders: The Wisdom of the World's Oldest People." went on a journey to find the oldest people in the world and document their histories.

His search took him to the United States, Italy, Portugal, Spain, Morocco, and Japan.

One of the supercentenarians interviewed by Friedman was Bettie Wilson (Born September 13, 1890, in New Albany, Mississippi, USA). Her parents were slaves that became sharecroppers after the Civil War. She was married and had three children, twelve grandchildren, forty-six great-grandchildren, ninety-five great-great-grandchildren, and forty great-great-great grandchildren". She clearly remembers "the long days of labor for her sharecropping family".

● ●

Emma Morano, an Italian supercentenarian (1899 – 2017) attributed her longevity to genetics, eating three raw eggs a day, and being single. She left her husband in 1938 because she didn´t want to be dominated by anyone.

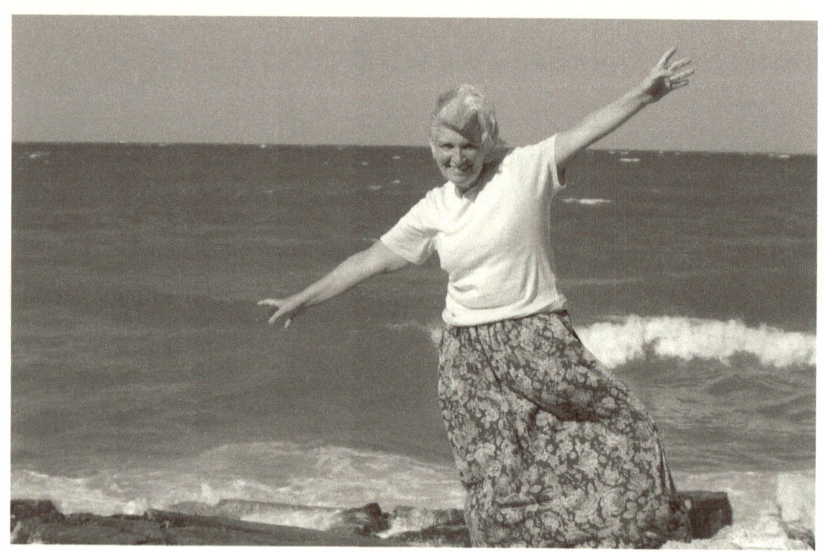

Summary

Some people seem to overcome all possible obstacles and be real winners in the race of life. These are the long-lived elderly, those who have successfully and healthily reached aging.

But what separates them from the common population? This is a question that science is still trying to answer.

Apparently, like everything in life, it takes a lot of effort.

This effort comes from a lifetime of good eating, healthy habits, and most of all, avoiding the temptation to succumb to bad habits.

A little push from genetics also seems to play a role, and who knows a little bit of luck? One day we'll find out.

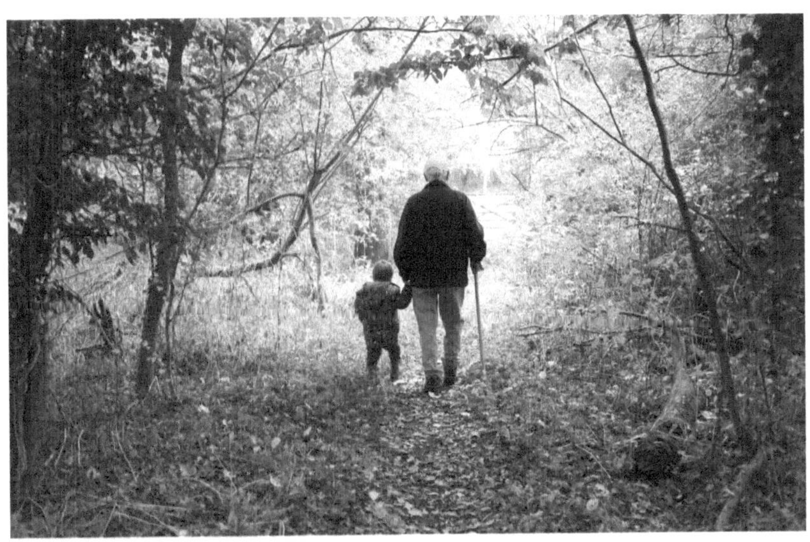

Author Bio

Valeri Chobanu

Founder & CEO at Chobanu Nutrition, Health Professional, Entrepreneur and Former Pro Athlete. NASM Certified Personal Trainer over 25 years experience, Health Coach, MMA Pro Competitor, Lifestyle Influencer and Nutrition Expert. Author and freelance writer of health, and fitness articles in the magazine Muscle & Fitness.

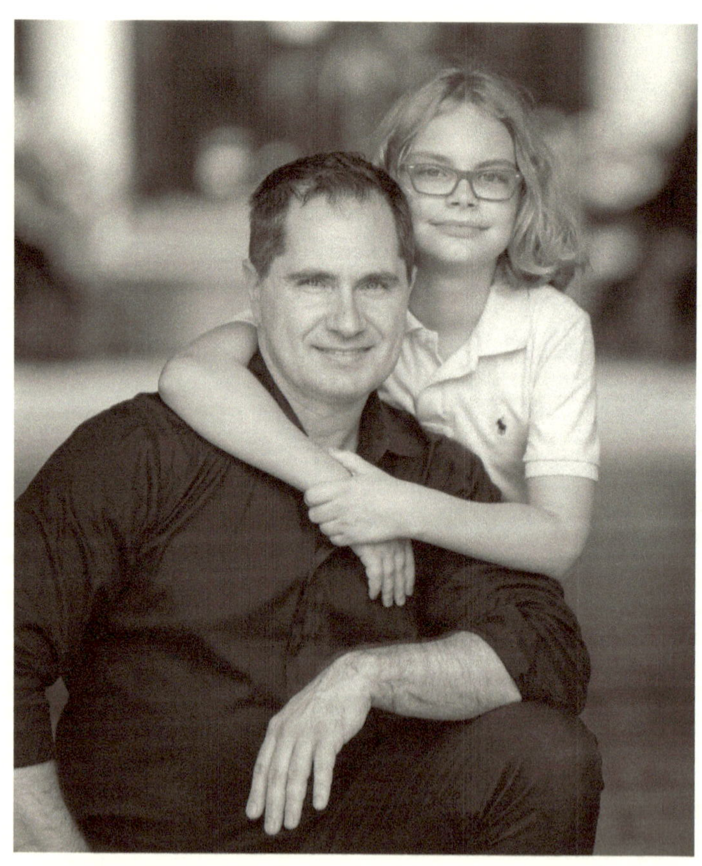

References

Caloric restriction and human longevity: what can we learn from the Okinawans? Willcox DC, Willcox BJ, Todoriki H, Curb JD, Suzuki M Biogerontology. 2006 Jun; 7(3):173-7.

Faye, Charlène, et al. "Neurobiological mechanisms of stress resilience and implications for the aged population." Current neuropharmacology 16.3 (2018): 234-270.

Fernandez-Mendoza, Julio, et al. "Objective short sleep duration increases the risk of all-cause mortality associated with possible vascular cognitive impairment." Sleep health 6.1 (2020): 71-78.

Field, Tiffany. "Yoga research review." Complementary therapies in clinical practice 24 (2016): 145-161.

https://www.apa.org/topics/resilience

https://www.nhs.uk/conditions/dementia/about/

https://www.nhs.uk/conditions/vitamins-and-minerals/

https://www.sleepfoundation.org/

Liguori, Ilaria, et al. "Oxidative stress, aging, and diseases." Clinical interventions in aging 13 (2018): 757.

McCay, Carl M., Mary F. Crowell, and Lewis A. Maynard. "The effect of retarded growth upon the length of life span and upon the ultimate body size: one figure." The journal of Nutrition 10.1 (1935): 63-79.

Mortality from circulatory diseases in Norway 1940-1945. STROM A, JENSEN RA. Lancet. 1951 Jan 20; 1(6647):126-9.

Pedersen, Bente Klarlund. "Which type of exercise keeps you young?." Current Opinion in Clinical Nutrition & Metabolic Care 22.2 (2019): 167-173.

Rathore, Mrithunjay, and Jessy Abraham. "Implication of asana, pranayama and meditation on telomere stability." International journal of yoga 11.3 (2018): 186.

Shlisky, Julie, et al. "Nutritional considerations for healthy aging and reduction in age-related chronic disease." Advances in Nutrition 8.1 (2017): 17.

Vidaček, Nikolina Škrobot, et al. "Telomeres, nutrition, and longevity: can we really navigate our aging?." The Journals of Gerontology: Series A 73.1 (2018): 39-47.

Weindruch, Richard. "Caloric restriction and aging." Scientific American 274.1 (1996): 46-52.

References

www.cancer.org

https://www.usa.gov/retirement

https://www.nia.nih.gov/health/aging-place-growing-older-home

https://www.nationalgeographic.com/books/features/5-blue-zones-where-the-worlds-healthiest-people-live/

https://www.bbc.com/news/world-europe-39610937

Mishra, Badri N. "Secret of eternal youth; Teaching from the centenarian hot spots ("blue zones")." Indian Journal of Community Medicine: Official Publication of Indian Association of Preventive & Social Medicine 34.4 (2009): 273.

Buettner, Dan. The blue zones: 9 lessons for living longer from the people who've lived the longest. National Geographic Books, 2012.

Max Roser, Esteban Ortiz-Ospina and Hannah Ritchie (2013) - "Life Expectancy". Published online at OurWorldInData.org. Retrieved from: https://ourworldindata.org/life-expectancy' [Online Resource]

Lister, Baron Joseph. "The classic: on the antiseptic principle in the practice of surgery." Clinical Orthopaedics and Related Research® 468.8 (2010): 2012-2016.

Gaynes, Robert. "The discovery of penicillin—new insights after more than 75 years of clinical use." Emerging Infectious Diseases 23.5 (2017): 849.

Desa, U. N. "World population prospects 2019: Highlights." New York (US): United Nations Department for Economic and Social Affairs (2019).

Foreman, Kyle J., et al. "Forecasting life expectancy, years of life lost, and all-cause and cause-specific mortality for 250 causes of death: reference and alternative scenarios for 2016–40 for 195 countries and territories." The Lancet 392.10159 (2018): 2052-2090.

Office for National Statistics. "Estimates of the Very Old (including centenarians)." (2016).

Medina, Lauren, Shannon Sabo, and Jonathan Vespa. Living Longer: Historical and Projected Life Expectancy in the United States, 1960 to 2060. US Department of Commerce, US Census Bureau, 2020

Avendano M, Glymour MM, Banks J, Mackenbach JP. Health disadvantage in US adults aged 50 to 74 years: A comparison of the health of rich and poor Americans with that of Europeans. American Journal of Public Health 2009; 99/3:540-548.

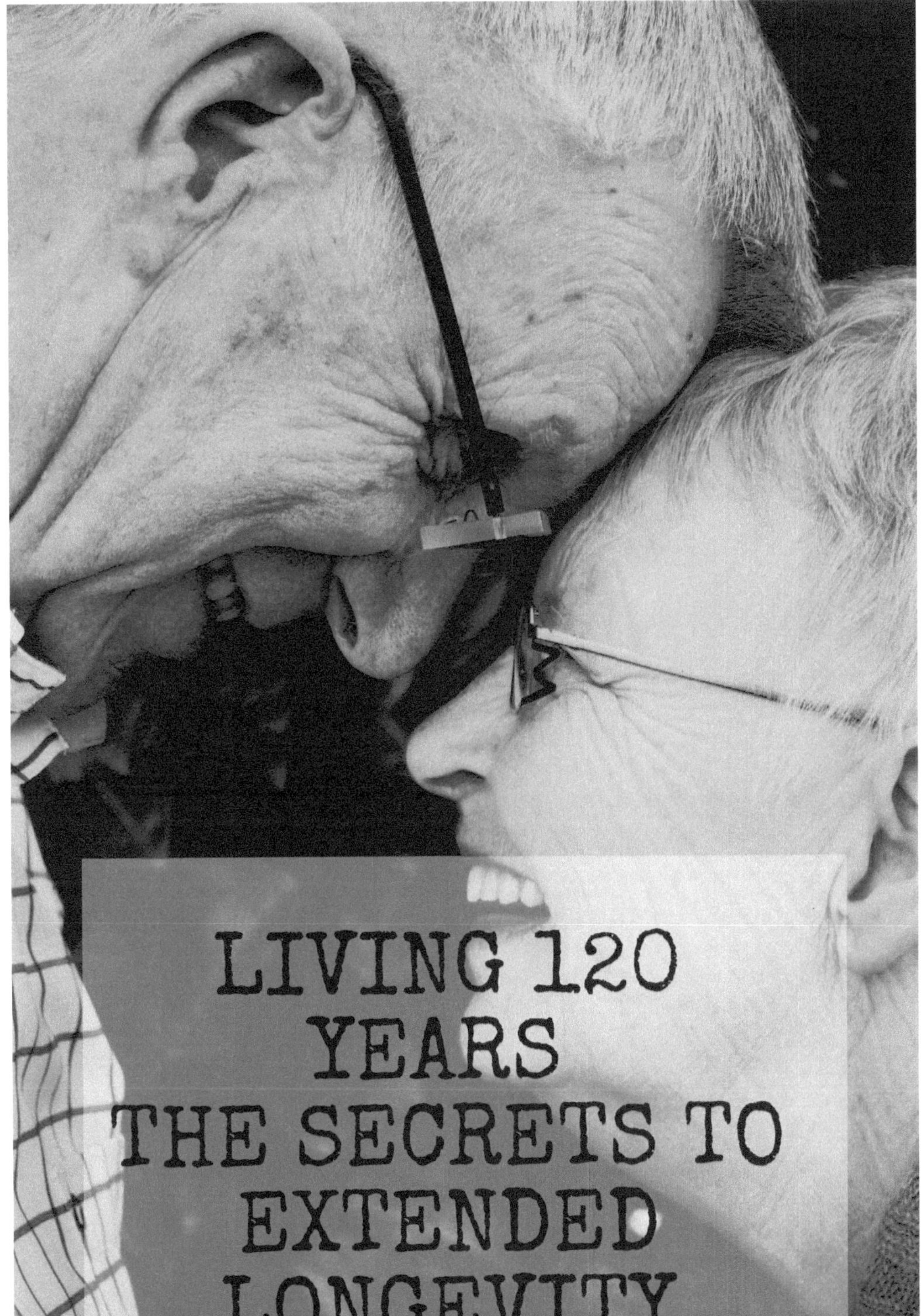

LIVING 120
YEARS
THE SECRETS TO
EXTENDED
LONGEVITY
www.chobanu.com